Extreme Weight Loss Hypnosis

A comprehensive guide on how to Develop Self Love, Confidence, Mindfulness& Healthy Eating Habits, Burn Fat + Hypnotic Gastric Band, Guided Meditations, Affirmations& Hypnosis

Elizabeth Collins

Table of Contents

Introduction

Hypnosis is rewiring your brain to add or to change your daily routine starting from your basic instincts. This happens due to the fact that while you are in a hypnotic state you are more susceptible to suggestions by the person who put you in this state. In the case of self-hypnosis, the person who made you enter the trance of hypnotism is yourself. Thus, the only person who can give you suggestions that can change your attitude in this method is you and you alone.

Again, you must forget the misconception that hypnosis is like sleeping because if it is then it would be impossible to give autosuggestions to yourself. Try to think about it like being in a very vivid daydream where you are capable of controlling every aspect of the situation you are in. This gives you the ability to change anything that may bother and hinder you to achieve the best possible result. If you are able to pull it off properly, then the possibility of improving yourself after a constant practice of the method will just be a few steps away.

Career

People say that motivation is the key to improve in your career. But no matter how you love your career, you must admit that there are aspects in your work that you really do not like doing. Even if it is a fact that you are good in the other tasks, there is that one duty that you dread. And every time you encounter this specific chore you seem to be slowed down and thus lessening your productivity at work. This is where self-hypnosis comes into play.

The first thing you need to do is find that task you do not like. In some cases there might be multiple of them depending on your personality and how you feel about your job. Now, try to look at why you do not like that task and do simple research on how to make the job a lot simpler. You can then start conditioning yourself to use the simple method every time you do the job.

After you are able to condition your state of mind to do the task, each time you encounter it will become the trigger for your trance and thus giving you the ability to perform it better. You will not be able to tell the difference since you will not mind it at all. Your coworkers and superiors though will definitely notice the change in your work style and in your productivity.

Family

It is easy to improve in a career. But to improve your relationship with your family can be a little tricky. Yet, self-hypnosis can still reprogram you to interact with your family members better by modifying how you react to the way they act. You will have the ability to adjust your way of thinking depending on the situation. This then allows you to respond in the most positive way possible, no matter how dreadful the scenario may be.

If you are in a fight with your husband/wife, for example, the normal reaction is to flare up and face fire with fire. The problem with this approach is it usually engulfs the entire relationship which might eventually lead up to separation. Being in a hypnotic state in this instance can help you think clearly and change the impulse of saying the words without thinking through. Anger will still be there, of course, that is the healthy way. But anger now under self-hypnosis can be channeled and stop being a raging inferno, you can turn it into a steady bonfire that can help you and your partner find common ground for whatever issue you are facing. The same applies in dealing with a sibling or children. If you are able to condition your mind to think more rationally or to get into the perspective of others, then you can have better family/friends' relationships.

Health and Physical Activities

Losing weight can be the most common reason why people will use self-hypnosis in terms of health and physical activities. But this is just one part of it. Self-hypnosis can give you a lot more to improve this aspect of your life. It works the same way while working out.

Most people tend to give up their exercise program due to the exhaustion they think they can no longer take. But through self-hypnosis, you will be able to tell yourself that the exhaustion is lessened and thus allowing you to finish the entire routine. Keep in mind though that your mind must never be conditioned to forget exhaustion, it must only not mind it until the end of the exercise. Forgetting it completely might lead you to not stopping to work out until your energy is depleted. It becomes counterproductive in this case.

Having a healthy diet can also be influenced by self-hypnosis. Conditioning your mind to avoid unhealthy food can be done. Thus, hypnosis will be triggered each you are tempted to eat a meal you are conditioned to consider as unhealthy. Your eating habit then can change to benefit you to improve your overall health.

Mental, Emotional and Spiritual Needs

Since self-hypnosis deals directly in how you think, it is then no secret that it can greatly improve your mental, emotional and spiritual needs. A clear mind can give your brain the ability to have more rational thoughts. Rationality then leads to better decision making and easy absorption and retention of information you might need to improve your mental capacity. You must set your expectations, though; this does not work like magic that can turn you into a genius. The process takes time depending on how far you want to go, how much you want to achieve. Thus, the effects will only be limited by how much you are able to condition your mind.

In terms of emotional needs, self-hypnosis cannot make you feel differently in certain situations. But it can condition you to take in each scenario a little lighter and make you deal with them better. Others think that getting rid of emotion can be the best course of action if you are truly able to rewire your brain. But they seem to forget that even though rational thinking is often influenced negatively by emotion, it is still necessary for you to decide on things basing on the common ethics and aesthetics of the real world. Self-hypnosis then can channel your emotion to work in a more positive way in terms of decision making and dealing with emotional hurdles and problems.

Spiritual need on the other hand is far easier to influence when it comes to doing self-hypnosis. As a matter of fact, most people with spiritual beliefs are able to do self-hypnosis each time they practice what they believe in. A deep prayer, for instance, is a way to self-hypnotize yourself to enter the trance to feel closer to a Divine existence. Chanting and meditation done by other religions also leads and have the same goal. Even the songs during a mass or praise and worship triggers self-hypnosis depending if the person allows them to do so.

Still, the improvements can only be achieved if you condition yourself that you are ready to accept them. The willingness to put an effort must also be there. An effortless hypnosis will only create the illusion that you are improving and thus will not give you the satisfaction of achieving your goal in reality.

How hypnosis can help resolve childhood issues

Another issue that hypnosis can help you with are problems from our past. If you have had traumatic situations from your childhood days, then you may have issues in all areas of your adult life. Unresolved issues from your past can lead to anxiety and depression in your later years. Childhood trauma is dangerous because it can alter many things in the brain both psychologically and chemically.

The most vital thing to remember about trauma from your childhood is that given a harmless and caring environment in which the child's vital needs for physical safety, importance, emotional security and attention are met, the damage that trauma and abuse cause can be eased and relieved. Safe and dependable relationships are also a dynamic component in healing the effects of childhood trauma in adulthood and make an atmosphere in which the brain can safely start the process of recovery.

Pure Hypnoanalysis is the lone most effective method of treatment available in the world today, for the resolution of phobias, anxiety, depression, fears, psychological and emotional problems/symptoms and eating disorders. It is a highly advanced form of hypnoanalysis (referred to as analytical hypnotherapy or hypno-analysis). Hypnoanalysis, in its numerous forms, is practiced all over the world; this method of hypnotherapy can completely resolve the foundation of anxieties in the unconscious mind, leaving the individual free of their symptoms for life.

There is a deeper realism active at all times around us and inside us. This reality commands that we must come to this world to find happiness, and every so often that our inner child stands in our way. This is by no means intentional; however, it desires to reconcile wounds from the past or address damaging philosophies which were troubling to us as children.

So disengaging the issues that upset us from earlier in our lives we have to find a way to bond with our internal child, we then need to assist in rebuilding this part of us which will, in turn, help us to be rid of all that has been hindering us from moving on.

Connecting with your inner child may seem like something

that may be hard or impossible to do, especially since they may be a part that has long been buried. It is a fairly easy exercise to do and can even be done right now. You will need about 20 minutes to complete this exercise. Here's what you do: find a quiet spot where you won't be disturbed and find pictures of you as a child if you think it may help.

Breathe in and loosen your clothing if you have to. Inhale deeply into your abdomen and exhale, repeat until you feel yourself getting relaxed; you may close your eyes and focus on getting less tense. Feel your forehead and head relax, let your face become relaxed and relax your shoulders. Allow your body to be limp and loose while you breathe slowly. Keep breathing slowly as you let all of your tension float away.

Now slowly count from 10 to 0 in your mind and try to think of a place from your childhood. The image doesn't have to be crystal clear right now but try to focus on exactly how you remember it and keep that image in mind. Imagine yourself as a child and imagine observing younger you; think about your clothes, expression, hair, etc. In your mind go and meet yourself, introduce yourself to you.

Chapter 1: How Does the Mind Work?

Your mind plays a critical role in helping you get healthy, get in shape, and stay that way. Your account is so vital that if you can't get your mind to cooperate with your body, you could be seriously undermining your chances of improving your overall health and wellbeing.

Often getting your head in line with your body is dependent on being able to make the most of your internal programming mechanism. In other words, what you tell yourself is vital to achieving anything you want. This self-talk can make, or break, your chances of becoming who you want to be.

For example, if you are continually telling yourself that you are not up to the task, that you are never going to make it, or that it is simply too hard to, then the chances of you not achieving your goals will be very slim. In contrast, if your self-talk is based upon your understanding of what it takes to be the best version of yourself, then the chances of you achieving anything that you want can explode through the roof. Best of all, you will give yourself a fighting chance when it comes to warding off any unwanted thoughts and feelings.

Also, it is vital to consider the fact that input from external sources can wreak havoc on your self-confidence and the way your mind process such data. You might get negative messages from people around you, or even attacks upon your choice of a healthy lifestyle. In some cases, attacks go to such extremes that some people stop talking to you, or decide not to hang out with you anymore, simply because you don't partake in eating or drinking binges.

These are people that you don't need in your life. It is best to surround yourself with like-minded people who will support you and help you in your endeavors. In doing so, you will be able to make better choices and stay on track.

Ultimately, you have the power to get on track and stay there. You don't need to depend on anything to help you make the most of your abilities to get in shape, drop some pounds and improve your overall health and wellbeing. Sure, it helps to be surrounded by supportive friends and family. But in the end, you have everything you need to be successful.

Throughout this the discussion presented, we are going to be looking at how you can summon that inner willpower that you have to aid you in making the most of any changes that you need to make... and help them stick. After all, anyone can go on one of those crash diets. But what will help you truly become what you want to be is your desire and willingness to make things happen. That coupled with a robust methodology, such as the power of meditation, you will come to develop your winning formula. You can think that this isn't a cookie-cutter solution. This is the type of approach which you can build for yourself. That means that what you do, what you choose to accomplish, and the way that you decide to do it will be your own particular way of doing things. That will surely guarantee that what you do will be both successful and sustainable.

With that in your back pocket, you can feel confident about moving on to bigger and better things in your life. You won't have to worry about being successful ever again simply because you have already achieved the most critical goal in your life. Based on that, you can begin to feel comfortable in your skin. And there is nothing better than feeling good about yourself while making the best of your opportunity to achieve everything that you have always wanted to achieve.

Chapter 2: What is Hypnosis?

Many psychiatrists have long considered hypnosis as a decent and respectable therapy method and it has become one of the regular psychiatric practices along with being showcased in Hollywood movies and poor illusion shows. Despite the general consensus, hypnosis is not an illusion, but it is a serious medical treatment if it is applied appropriately. Its helpfulness is undeniable; however, it can also be hazardous. Why? Because in some regards, hypnosis is a kind of mind control technique. Furthermore, hypnosis is sometimes still recognized to be some mysterious phenomenon, or more 'rational' people simply view it as a trick. The 'enlightened' scientific version of the latter opinion claims that the hypnotized subject almost always tries to meet the expectations of the hypnotist; therefore, the hypnotic phenomena are nothing more than role-playing.

What is the truth about hypnosis?

What if hypnosis isn't just the tricky deception we see at shows? The truth is that hypnosis is closely connected to meditation. Hypnosis uses techniques of deep breathing and puts the subject into an incredibly powerful relaxed state in order to make them open to suggestions. This psychiatric technique does not apply the usage of a pendulum in front of a person's eyes, as is commonly believed. What it does is to create a relaxed atmosphere so that the patient can feel comfortable and trust in their therapist. The purpose is to be able to reach the patient at different conscious levels so that they can be more open to suggestions.

How did hypnosis originate?

Theories suggest that people may have used hypnosis as early as prehistoric times. The rites of worship and shamanism are partly explained by self-suggestion. It was presumably discovered accidentally through religious activities such as meditation, cult activities, and rituals. The first figures, most likely about hypnosis, have survived from ancient Egypt. The oldest description is on an Egyptian papyrus roll from 3766 BC: "Put your hand on the arm to relieve the pain and say that the pain has ceased." The Westcar papyrus preserved at the Neues Museum in Berlin reports that Jaya-manekh had persuaded a very wild lion to obey him. This source undoubtedly indicates that animal hypnosis was already known and practiced in Egypt. They may have known about hypnosis utilized with humans. Along with Jaya-manekh,

Deda also used animal hypnosis, though he only presented his evidence using ducks, geese and an ox (Mongiovi, 2014).

The roots of what we now call hypnosis must be found at the end of the Middle Ages and in modern times.

In the sixteenth century, Paracelsus hypothesized about the devious relationship between celestial bodies and the human body. He considered it important to use various mineral medicines in addition to the proper magic spells. This laid the foundation for the theory of "mineral magnetism." Franz Anton Mesmer (1720-1815) adopted and continued the principle of magnetic effect. Through his group healings in a spectacular séance (reminiscent of the exorcism ceremony in its outward appearance), he became well-known for being the founder of the first hypnosis school. Nonetheless, in practice, verbal suggestion was lacking. He attributed therapeutic efficacy to the mysterious "magnetic fluid" that could be transmitted to the patient by hand movement ("magnetic passage") over the patient's body. He explained this with animated magnetism ('magnetismus animalis'; the magnetism of breathing, soul-like creatures) and placed magnets on the patients. Because of its popularity, hypnosis has long been called mesmerization (Rose, 2017).

Many others later criticized Mesmer. For example, Alfred Russel Wallace explained hypnosis with a phrenological map, and Friedrich Engels hypnotized a 12-year-old boy without a magnet. Mesmer was a pupil of the Marquis Armand-Marc-Jacques de Chastenet Puitureur (1721-1825). He initially accepted his master's theory, but his practice, unlike Mesmer's, lacked spectacular elements. His patients, who were subjected to verbal suggestions, behaved similarly to sleepwalkers and called their condition provocative somnambulism (Mongiovi, 2014).

If you've watched some of the old western movies, you may have noticed that alcohol was utilized as an anesthetic in operations. A few hundred years ago, if someone's arm had to be amputated, the patient would have been given a cheap whiskey for numbing purposes because they didn't have the luxury of using medicines like today. But alcohol wasn't the only anesthetic method. Hypnosis was also used for similar reasons to relieve pain in order to prevent subjects from entering neurogenic shock in the 1800s. If you really think about it, this was a very useful method. One of the best examples of the use of hypnosis in surgery is James Esdaile, a Scottish doctor who applied the method to more than 3000 patients in India with superior accomplishment (Spiegel, 2007).

In the 19th century, France took the lead in hypnosis research with centers such as Nancy (Ambroise-Auguste Liebeault, Hippolyte Bernheim) and Paris (Jean-Martin Charcot).

Sigmund Freud visited Jean-Martin Charcot in Paris in 1885, observing Mesmer's method and trying it out for himself. This became the starting point for his studies on hysteria. He later abandoned this method and switched to free association. It is clear from his writings that he continued to deal with hypnosis. Oskar Vogt (1870-1959) and his student Johannes Heinrich Schultz (1884-1970) researched and developed autogenous training from German hypnosis. Later Klaus Thomas did research as well. The main researchers in America were Milton H. Erickson (indirect hypnosis), and Kroger and Dave Elman (authorial hypnosis). John Hartland is the best-known hypnotist in the UK. His book, the Dictionary of Medical and Dental Hypnosis, is still the official textbook for British hypnotists. Milton H. Erickson developed the method of hypnotherapy, from which several psychological techniques were improved.

Can anyone be hypnotized?

Hypnosis is an unpredictable state. You may be easily hypnotized, while it won't work for others. It is still a mystery to psychiatrists and neuroscientists how hypnosis works. The only thing we know is that it can work, but we don't have any idea how it works. A scientific study on the mechanism of hypnosis researched why some people are more responsive to hypnosis than others. As reported by the research, an individual's hypnotizability is more easily linked to brain function and the capability of connection. According to the study, the relationships between the left dorsolateral prefrontal cortex and the brain areas that treat the information are more effective than those of other subjects (Hoeft, Gabrieli, Whitfield-Gabrieli, Haas, Bammer, Menon, & Spiegel, 2013). Dr. Clifford N. Lazarus says that the individual must be willing and open to hypnosis; otherwise, it doesn't work: "Contrary to popular belief, people under hypnosis are in total control of themselves and would never do anything they would normally find highly objectionable" (Lazarus, 2013). It implies that if you don't want to be hypnotized, you can resist.

What occurs during hypnotism?

Imagine that you are watching an exciting action movie. A dangerous group chases the main character. The protagonist is trapped in a building, and the bad guys are waiting for him outside. You have been immersed in the movie when one of your family members asks you to give them a pillow. What do you do? I suppose you will take the pillow and give it to your relative without taking your eyes off the screen. When you are hypnotized, a similar scenario occurs. You focus on the matter intensely, and everything else becomes irrelevant. The greater the focus, the stronger the tendency to follow the suggestions of the therapist.

However, there is a tiny difference between the attention paid during a movie and in hypnosis. People who watch movies profoundly are more inclined not to reply to the questions they are asked; however, the opposite occurs during hypnosis. Why is that? Based on the observation of Freudian psychologists, this happens due to the difference between the phases of human awareness. They believe that there are three layers of human consciousness: preconsciousness, consciousness, and the unconscious level. These levels are depicted with an analogy. The level of consciousness that is compared to the visible part of an iceberg seeing it from the water surface represents the moments of our awareness about what's happening around us when we are awake (Cherry, 2019).

The iceberg's water level represents the level of preconsciousness and illustrates what we can't remember at the very moment but can recall if we want to. For instance, when you need to go somewhere that you have been before but don't remember the way, you will still find the right street. How is it possible? Because your preconsciousness level provides you with the necessary information to easily find the way you don't remember. You don't store this information in the level of consciousness. The part which is underwater and has the most massive volume is associated with the unconscious level in the iceberg analogy. We store fears, irrational and unacceptable desires, and deep convictions at the unconscious level. In order to bring them to the surface, we use hypnosis which can touch this level of our awareness. In the unconscious phase, right or wrong, moral or immoral don't exist because the filter system, which directs a person's ordinary life, is disabled, and our capacity for analyzing matters is discharged. In this level of consciousness, our deepest desires come true. However, unlike in a dream, our ability to perceive danger is still alert during hypnosis which means if the individual fears hypnosis or considers it dangerous, they won't allow the therapist to reach that phase of awareness (Journal Psyche, n. d.).

Can we really recall the hidden parts of our past under hypnosis?

Many therapists think that unsolved dilemmas or issues in the past are transmitted to the future, confusing people and producing psychological disorders. Therapists use the method of hypnosis to make their patients remember their past lives and release 'emotional baggage'. However, we need to know that memory is in an unstable form in the hypnotic subconscious. Therefore, hypnosis can cause a person to think that they are experiencing an event that hasn't occurred in real life. Hence, many experts reject the thesis that details are remembered, as they can be easily distorted. But it also means that we can alter our negative memories and convictions and exchange them with favorable ones (Thompson, n. d.).

Is hypnosis a biological phenomenon?

Research suggests that hypnosis has a biological aspect because of an electrical impulse between our brain cells. Cells send these impulses synchronously in groups and they don't isolate them. Also, various phases of consciousness have different frequencies (brain wave rhythm). If we acknowledge the electrical impulses as the language of the brain, we can pretend that different frequencies communicate at different speeds. These different speeds are called Alpha, Beta, Theta and Delta.

When we are asleep, the brain waves slow down and produce the so-called delta frequency waves. When it reveals relatively higher frequency vigilance, this is called beta frequency waves. Research has shown that brain waves are at theta frequency during hypnosis. In the theta frequency, there is both a level of subconscious awareness as well as a high concentration in sleep. It has been noticed that theta frequency occurs more frequently in the brains of people who are more susceptible to hypnosis. Besides, some researchers claim that hypnotizability is inherited and strongly conditioned by the presence of specific genes (Adachi, Jensen, Lee, Miró, Osman, Tomé-Pires, 2016).

Chapter 3: How Hypnosis Can Help You Lose Weight

Losing weight with hypnosis works just like any other change with hypnosis will. However, it is important to understand the step-by-step process so that you know exactly what to expect during your weight loss journey with the support of hypnosis. In general, there are about seven steps that are involved with weight loss using hypnosis. The first step is when you decide to change; the second step involves your sessions; the third and fourth are your changed mindset and behaviors, the fifth step involves your regressions, the sixth is your management routines, and the seventh is your lasting change. To give you a better idea of what each of these parts of your journey looks like, let's explore them in greater detail below.

In your first step toward achieving weight loss with hypnosis, you have decided that you desire change and that you are willing to try hypnosis as a way to change your approach to weight loss. At this point, you are aware of the fact that you want to lose weight, and you have been shown the possibility of losing weight through hypnosis. You may find yourself feeling curious, open to trying something new, and a little bit skeptical as to whether or not this is actually going to work for you. You may also be feeling frustrated, overwhelmed, or even defeated by the lack of success you have seen using other weight loss methods, which may be what lead you to seek out hypnosis in the first place. At this stage, the best thing you can do is practice keeping an open and curious mind, as this is how you can set yourself up for success when it comes to your actual hypnosis sessions.

Your sessions account for stage two of the process. Technically, you are going to move from stage two through to stage five several times over before you officially move into stage six. Your sessions are the stage where you actually engage in hypnosis, nothing more and nothing less. During your sessions, you need to maintain your open mind and stay focused on how hypnosis can help you. If you are struggling to stay open-minded or are still skeptical about how this might work, you can consider switching from absolute confidence that it will help to have a curiosity about how it might help instead.

Following your sessions, you are first going to experience a changed mindset. This is where you start to feel far more confident in your ability to lose weight and in your ability to keep the weight off. At first, your mindset may still be shadowed by doubt, but as you continue to use hypnosis and see your results, you will realize that it is entirely possible for you to create success with hypnosis. As these pieces of evidence start to show up in your own life, you will find your hypnosis sessions becoming even more powerful and even more successful.

In addition to a changed mindset, you are going to start to see changed behaviors. They may be smaller at first, but you will find that they increase over time until they reach the point where your behaviors reflect exactly the lifestyle you have been aiming to have. The best part about these changed behaviors is that they will not feel forced, nor will they feel like you have had to encourage yourself to get here: your changed mindset will make these changed behaviors incredibly easy for you to choose. As you continue working on your hypnosis and experiencing your changed mind, you will find that your behavioral changes grow more significant and more effortless every single time.

Following your hypnosis and your experiences with changed mindset and behaviors, you are likely going to experience regression periods. Regression periods are characterized by periods of time where you begin to engage in your old mindset and behavior once again. This happens because you have experienced this old mindset and behavioral patterns so many times over that they continue to have deep roots in your subconscious mind. The more you uproot them and reinforce your new behaviors with consistent hypnosis sessions, the more success you will have in eliminating these old behaviors and replacing them entirely with new ones. Anytime you experience the beginning of a regression period; you should set aside some time to engage in a hypnosis session to help you shift your mindset back into the state that you want and need it to be in.

Your management routines account for the sixth step, and they come into place after you have effectively experienced a significant and lasting change from your hypnosis practices. At this point, you are not going to need to schedule as frequent of hypnosis sessions because you are experiencing such significant changes in your mindset. However, you may still want to do hypnosis sessions on a fairly consistent basis to ensure that your mindset remains changed and that you do not revert into old patterns. Sometimes, it can take up to 3-6 months or longer with these consistent management routine hypnosis sessions to maintain your changes and prevent you from experiencing a significant regression in your mindset and behavior.

 The final step in your hypnosis journey is going to be the step where you come upon lasting changes. At this point, you are unlikely to need to schedule hypnosis sessions any longer. You should not need to rely on hypnosis at all to change your mindset because you have experienced such significant changes already, and you no longer find yourself regressing into old behaviors. With that being said, you may find that from time to time, you need to have a hypnosis session just to maintain your changes, particularly when an unexpected trigger may arise that may cause you to want to regress your behaviors. These unexpected changes can happen for years following your successful changes, so staying on top of them and relying on your healthy coping method of hypnosis is important as it will prevent you from experiencing a significant regression later in life.

Using Hypnosis to Encourage Healthy Eating and Discourage Unhealthy Eating

As you go through using hypnosis to support you with weight loss, there are a few ways that you are going to do so. One of the ways is, obviously, to focus on weight loss itself. Another way, however, is to focus on topics surrounding weight loss. For example, you can use hypnosis to help you encourage yourself to eat healthy while also helping discourage yourself from unhealthy eating. Effective hypnosis sessions can help you bust cravings for foods that are going to sabotage your success while also helping you feel more drawn to making choices that are going to help you effectively lose weight.

Many people will use hypnosis as a way to change their cravings, improve their metabolism, and even help themselves acquire a taste for eating healthier foods. You may also use this to help encourage you to develop the motivation and energy to actually prepare healthier foods and eat them so that you are more likely to have these healthier options available for you. If cultivating the motivation for preparing and eating healthy foods has been problematic for you, this type of hypnosis focus can be incredibly helpful.

Using Hypnosis to Encourage Healthy Lifestyle Changes

In addition to helping you encourage yourself to eat healthier while discouraging yourself from eating unhealthy foods, you can also use hypnosis to help encourage you to make healthy lifestyle changes. This can support you with everything from exercising more frequently to picking up more active hobbies that support your wellbeing in general.

You may also use this to help you eliminate hobbies or experiences from your life that may encourage unhealthy dietary habits in the first place. For example, if you tend to binge eat when you are stressed out, you might use hypnosis to help you navigate stress more effectively so that you are less likely to binge eat when you are feeling stressed out. If you tend to eat when you are feeling emotional or bored, you can use hypnosis to help you change those behaviors, too.

Hypnosis can be used to change virtually any area of your life that motivates you to eat unhealthily or otherwise neglect self-care to the point where you are sabotaging yourself from healthy weight loss. It truly is an incredibly versatile practice that you can rely on that will help you with weight loss, as well as help you with creating a healthier lifestyle in general. With hypnosis, there are countless ways that you can improve the quality of your life, making it an incredibly helpful practice for you to rely on.

The Benefits of Hypnotherapy for Weight Loss

It is hard to pinpoint the single best benefit that comes from using hypnosis as a way to engage in weight loss. Hypnosis is a natural, lasting, and deeply impactful weight loss habit that you can use to completely change the way you approach weight loss, and food in general, for the rest of your life.

With hypnosis, you are not ingesting anything that results in hypnosis working. Instead, you are simply listening to guided hypnosis meditations that help you transform the way your subconscious mind works. As you change the way your subconscious mind works, you will find yourself not even having cravings or unhealthy food urges in the first place. This means no more fighting against your desires, yo-yo dieting, "falling off the wagon," or experiencing any inner conflict around your eating patterns, or your weight loss exercises that are helping you lose the weight. Instead, you will begin to have an entirely new mindset and perspective around weight loss that leads to you having more success in losing weight and keeping it off for good.

In addition to hypnosis itself being effective, you can also combine hypnosis with any other weight loss strategy you are using. Changed dietary behaviors, exercise routines, any medications you may be taking with the advisement of your medical practitioner, and any other weight loss practices you may be engaging in can all safely be done with hypnosis. By including hypnosis in your existing weight loss routines, you can improve your effectiveness and rapidly increase the success you experience in your weight loss patterns.

Finally, hypnosis can be beneficial for many things beyond weight loss. One of the side effects that you will probably notice once you start using hypnosis to help change your weight loss experience is that you also experience a boost in your confidence, self-esteem, and general feelings of positivity. Many people who use hypnosis on a regular basis find themselves feeling more positive and in better spirits in general. This means that not only will you lose weight, but you will also feel incredible and will have a happy and positive mood as well.

Chapter 4: What is Self-Hypnosis?

If you can afford to undergo a series of hypnotherapy sessions with a specialist, you may do so. This is ideal as you will work with a professional who can guide you through the treatment and will also provide you with valuable advice on nutrition and exercises.

Clinical Hypnotherapy

When first meeting with a therapist, they start by explaining to you the type of hypnotherapy he or she is using. Then you will discuss your personal goals so the therapist can better understand your motivations.

The formal session will start with your therapist, speaking in a gentle and soothing voice. This will help you relax and feel safe during the entire therapy.

Once your mind is more receptive, the therapist will start suggesting ways that can help you modify your exercise or eating habits as well as other ways to help you reach your weight loss goals.

Specific words or repetition of particular phrases can help

you at this stage. The therapist may also help you in visualizing the body image you want, which is one effective technique in hypnotherapy.

To end the session, the therapist will bring you out from the hypnotic stage, and you will start to be more alert. Your personal goals will influence the duration of the hypnotherapy sessions as well as the number of total sessions that you may need. Most people begin to see results in as few as two to four sessions.

DIY Hypnotherapy

If you are not comfortable working with a professional hypnotherapist or you can't afford the sessions, you can choose to perform self-hypnosis. While this is not as effective as the sessions under a professional, you can still try it and see if it can help you with your weight loss goals.

HERE ARE THE STEPS IF YOU WISH TO PRACTICE SELF-HYPNOSIS:

Believe in the power of hypnotism. Remember, this alternative treatment requires the person to be open and willing. It will not work for you if your mind is already set against it.

Find a comfortable and quiet room to practice hypnotherapy. Ideally, you should find a place that is free from noise and where no one can disturb you. Wear loose clothes and set relaxing music to help in setting up the mood.

Find a focal point. Choose an object in a room that you can focus on. Use your concentration on this object so you can start clearing your mind of all thoughts.

Breathe deeply. Start with five deep breaths, inhaling through your nose and exhaling through your mouth.

Close your eyes. Think about your eyelids becoming heavy and just let them close slowly.

Imagine that all stress and tension are coming out of your body. Let this feeling move down from your head, to your shoulders, to your chest, to your arms, to your stomach, to your legs, and finally to your feet.

Clear your mind. When you are relaxed, your account must be clear, and you can initiate the process of self-hypnotism.

Visualize a pendulum. In your mind, picture a moving swing. The movement of the pendulum is popular imagery used in hypnotism to encourage focus.

Start visualizing your ideal body image and size. This should help you instill in your subconscious the importance of a healthy diet and exercise.

Suggest to yourself to avoid unhealthy food and start exercising regularly. You can use a particular mantra such as "I will exercise at least three times a week. Unhealthy food will make me sick."

Wake up. Once you have achieved what you want during hypnosis, you must wake yourself. Start by counting back from one to 10 and wake up when you reach 10.

Remember, a healthy diet doesn't mean that you have to reduce your food intake significantly. Just cut your consumption of food that is not healthy for you. Never hypnotize yourself out of eating. Only suggest to yourself to eat less of the food that you know is just making you fat.

Chapter 5: Hypnosis and Weight Loss

Hypnosis plays a vital role in medicinal solutions. In modern-day society, it is recommended for treating many different conditions, including obesity or weight loss in individuals who are overweight. It also serves patients who have undergone surgery exceptionally well, mainly if they are restricted from exercising after surgery. Given that it is the perfect option for losing weight, it is additionally helpful to anyone who is disabled or recovering from an injury.

Once you understand the practice and how it is conducted, you will find that everything makes sense. Hypnosis works for weight loss because of the relationship between our minds and bodies. Without proper communication being relayed from our minds to our bodies, we would not be able to function correctly. Since hypnosis allows the brain to adopt new ideas and habits, it can help push anyone in the right direction and could potentially improve our quality of living.

Adopting new habits can help eliminate fear, improve confidence, and inspire you to maintain persistence and a sense of motivation on your weight loss journey. Since two of the most significant issue's society faces today are media-based influences and a lack of motivation, you can quickly solve any problems related by merely correcting your mind.

Correcting your mind is an entirely different mission on its own, or without hypnosis, that is. It is a challenge that most will get frustrated. Nobody wants to deal with themselves. Although that may be true, perhaps one of the best lessons hypnosis teaches you is the significance of spending time focusing on your intentions. Daily practicing of hypnosis includes focusing on specific ideas. Once these ideas are normalized in your daily routine and life, you will find it easier to cope with struggles and ultimately break bad habits, which is the ultimate goal.

In reality, it takes 21 consecutive days to break a bad habit, but only if a person remains persistent, integrating both a conscious and consistent effort to quit or rectify a practice. It takes the same amount of time to adopt a new healthy habit. With hypnosis, it can take up to three months to either break a bad habit or form a new one. However, even though hypnosis takes longer, it tends to work far more effectively than just forcing yourself to do something you don't want to do.

Our brains are robust operating systems that can be fooled under the right circumstances. Hypnosis has been proven to be useful for breaking habits and adopting new ones due to its powerful effect on the mind. It can be measured in the same line of consistency and power as affirmations. Now, many would argue that hypnosis is unnecessary and that completing a 90-day practice of hypnotherapy to change habits for weight loss is a complete waste of time. However, when you think about someone who needs to lose weight but can't seem to do it, then you might start reconsidering it as a helpful solution to the problem. It's no secret that the human brain requires far more than a little push or single affirmation to thrive. Looking at motivational video clips and reading quotes every day is great, but is it helping you to move further than from A to B?

It's true that today, we are faced with a sense of rushing through life. Asking an obese or unhealthy individual why they gained weight, there's a certainty that you'll receive similar answers.

Could it be that no one has time to, for instance, cook or prep healthy meals, visit the gym or move their bodies? Apart from making up excuses as to why you can't do something, there's actual evidence hidden in the reasons why we sell ourselves short and opt for the easy way out.

Could it be that the majority of individuals have just become lazy?

Regardless of your excuses, reasons or inabilities, hypnosis debunks the idea that you have to go all out to get healthier. Losing weight to improve your physical appearance has always been a challenge, and although there is no easy way out, daily persistence and 10 to 60 minutes a day of practice could help you to lose weight. Not just that, but it can also restructure your brain and help you to develop better habits, which will guide you in experiencing a much more positive and sustainable means of living.

Regardless of the practice or routine, you follow at the end of the day, the principle of losing weight always remains the same. You have to follow a balanced diet in proportion with a sustainable exercise routine.

By not doing so is where most people tend to go wrong with their weight loss journeys. It doesn't matter whether it's a diet supplement, weight loss tea, or even hypnosis. Your diet and exercise routine still play an increasingly important role in losing weight and will be the number one factor that will help you to obtain permanent results. There's a lot of truth in the advice given that there aren't any quick fixes to help you lose weight faster than what's recommended. Usually, anything that promotes standard weight loss, which is generally about two to five pounds a week, depending on your current Body Mass Index (BMI), works no matter what it is. The trick to losing weight doesn't necessarily lie in what you do, but instead in how you do it.

When people start with hypnosis, they may be very likely to quit after a few days or weeks, as it may not seem useful or it isn't leading to any noticeable results.

Nevertheless, if you remain consistent with it, eat a balanced diet instead of crash dieting, and follow a simple exercise routine, then you will find that it has a lot more to offer you than just weight loss. Even though weight loss is the ultimate goal, it's essential to keep in mind that lasting results don't occur overnight. There are no quick fixes, especially with hypnosis.

Adopting the practice, you will discover many benefits, yet two of the most important ones are healing and learning how to activate the fat burning process inside of your body.

Hypnosis is not a diet, nor is it a fast track method to get you where you want to go. Instead, it is a tool used to help individuals reach their goals by implementing proper habits. These habits can help you achieve results by focusing on appropriate diet and exercise. Since psychological issues influence most weight-related issues, hypnosis acts as the perfect tool, laying a foundation for a healthy mind.

Hypnosis is not a type of mind control, yet it is designed to alter your mind by shifting your feelings toward liking something that you might have hated before, such as exercise or eating a balanced diet. The same goes for quitting sugar or binge eating. Hypnosis identifies the root of the issues you may be dealing with and works by rectifying it accordingly. Given that it changes your thought pattern, you may also experience a much calmer and relaxed approach to everything you do.

Hypnosis works by maintaining changes made in mind because of neuroplasticity. Consistent hypnotherapy sessions create new patterns in the brain that result in the creation of new habits. Since consistency is the number one key to losing weight, it acts as a solution to overcome barriers in your mind, which is something the majority of individuals struggle. Hypnosis can also provide you with many techniques to meet different goals, such as gastric band hypnosis, which works by limiting eating habits, causing you to refrain from overeating.

Chapter 6: The Power of Affirmations

Today is another day. Today is a day for you to start making a euphoric, satisfying life. Today is the day to begin to discharge every one of your impediments. Today is the day for you to get familiar with the privileged insights of life. You can transform yourself into improving things. You, as of now, include the devices inside you to do as such. These devices are your considerations and your convictions.

What Are Positive Affirmations?

For those of you who aren't acquainted with the advantages of positive affirmations, I'd prefer to clarify a little about them. A statement is genuinely anything you state or think. A great deal of what we typically report and believe is very harmful and doesn't make great encounters for us. We need to retrain our reasoning and to talk into positive examples if we need to change us completely.

An affirmation opens the entryway. It's a starting point on the way to change. When I talk about doing affirmations, I mean deliberately picking words that will either help take out something from your life or help make something new in your life.

Each idea you think and each word you express is an affirmation. The entirety of our self-talk, our interior exchange, is a flood of oaths. You're utilizing statements each second, whether you know it or not. You're insisting and making your background with each word and thought.

Your convictions are just routine reasoning examples that you learned as a youngster. The vast numbers of them work very well for you. Different beliefs might be restricting your capacity to make the very things you state you need. What you need and what you trust your merit might be unusual. You have to focus on your contemplations with the goal that you can start to dispose of the ones making encounters you don't need in your life.

It would help if you understood that each grievance is an affirmation of something you figure you don't need in your life. Each time you blow up, you're asserting that you need more annoyance in your life. Each time you feel like a casualty, you're confirming that you need to keep on feeling like a casualty. If you believe that you think that life isn't giving you what you need in your reality, at that point, it's sure that you will never have the treats that experience provides for others that is until you change how you think and talk.

You're not a terrible individual for intuition, how you do. You've quite recently never figured out how to think and talk. Individuals all through the world are quite recently starting to discover that our contemplations make our encounters. Your folks most likely didn't have the foggiest idea about this, so they couldn't in any way, shape, or form instruct it to you. They showed you what to look like at life in the manner that their folks told them. So, no one isn't right. In any case, it's the ideal opportunity for us all to wake up and start to deliberately make our lives in a manner that satisfies and bolsters us. You can do it. I can do it. We, as a whole, can do it, we need to figure out how. So how about we get to it?

I'll talk about affirmations as a rule, and afterwards, I'll get too specific everyday issues and tell you the best way to roll out positive improvements in your wellbeing, your funds, your affection life, etc. Once you figure out how to utilize affirmations, at that point, you can apply the standards in all circumstances. A few people say that "affirmations don't work" (which is an affirmation in itself) when what they mean is that they don't have a clue how to utilize them accurately. Some of the time, individuals will say their affirmations once per day and gripe the remainder of the time. It will require some investment for affirmations to work if they're done that way. The grumbling affirmations will consistently win, because there is a higher amount of them, and they're generally said with extraordinary inclination.

In any case, saying affirmations is just a piece of the procedure. What you wrap up of the day and night is significantly progressively significant. The key to having your statements work rapidly and reliably is to set up air for them to develop in. Affirmations resemble seeds planted in soil: poor soil, poor development. Fertile soil, bottomless event. The more you decide to think contemplations that cause you to feel great, the faster the affirmations work.

So, think upbeat musings, it's that straightforward. What's more, it is feasible. How you decide to believe at present is only a decision. You may not understand it since you've thought along these lines for such a long time, yet it truly is a decision. Presently, today, this second, you can decide to change your reasoning. Your life won't pivot for the time being. Yet, in case you're reliable and settle on the decision regularly to think considerations that cause you to feel great, you'll unquestionably roll out positive improvements in each part of your life.

Positive Affirmations and How to Use Them

Positive affirmations are positive articulations that depict an ideal circumstance, propensity, or objective that you need to accomplish. Rehashing regularly these positive explanations, influences the psyche brain profoundly, and triggers it without hesitation, to bring what you are reworking into the real world.

The demonstration of rehashing the affirmations, intellectually or so anyone might hear, inspires the individual reworking them, builds the desire and inspiration, and pulls in open doors for development and achievement.

This demonstration likewise programs the psyche to act as per the rehashed words, setting off the inner mind-brain to take a shot at one's sake, to offer the positive expressions materialize.

Affirmations are extremely valuable for building new propensities, rolling out positive improvements throughout one's life, and for accomplishing objectives.

Affirmations help in weight misfortune, getting progressively engaged, concentrating better, changing propensities, and accomplishing dreams.

They can be helpful in sports, in business, improving one's

wellbeing, weight training, and in numerous different zones.

These positive articulations influence in a proper manner, the body, the brain, and one's sentiments

Rehashing affirmations is very reasonable. Despite this, a lot of people do not know about this truth. Individuals, for the most part, restate negative statements, not positive ones. This is called negative self-talk.

On the off chance that you have been disclosing to yourself how miserable you can't contemplate, need more cash, or how troublesome life is, you have been rehashing negative affirmations.

Along these lines, you make more challenges and more issues, since you are concentrating on the problems, and in this way, expanding them, rather than concentrating on the arrangements.

A great many people rehash in their psyches pessimistic words and proclamations concerning the contrary circumstances and occasions in their lives, and therefore, make progressively bothersome circumstances.

Words work in two different ways, to assemble or obliterate. It is how we use them that decides if they will bring tremendous or destructive outcomes.

Affirmations in Modern Times

It is said that the French analyst and drug specialist Emile Coue is the individual who carried this subject to the open's consideration in the mid-twentieth century.

Emile Coue saw that when he told his patients how viable an elixir was, the outcomes were superior to if he didn't utter a word. He understood that musings that consume our psyches become a reality and that rehashing concepts and considerations is a sort of autosuggestion.

Emile Coue is associated with his acclaimed proclamation, "Consistently, all around, I am showing signs of improvement and better."

Later in the twentieth century, this was Louise Hay, who concentrated on this point and called autosuggestion affirmations.

Chapter 7: 100 Positive Affirmations for Weight Loss

George taught Bonnie a hundred useful positive affirmations for weight loss and to keep her motivated. She chose the ones that she wanted to build in her program and used them every day. Bonnie was losing weight very slowly, which bothered her very much. She thought she was going in the wrong direction and was about to give up, but George told her not to worry because it was a completely natural speed. It takes time for the subconscious to collate all the information and start working according to her conscious will. Besides, her body remembered the fast weight loss, but her subconscious remembered her emotional damage, and now it is trying to prevent it. In reality, after some months of hard work, she started to see the desired results. She weighed 74 kilos (163 lbs.).

According to dietitians, the success of dieting is greatly influenced by how people talk about lifestyle changes for others and themselves.

The use of "I should," or "I must" is to avoid whenever possible. Anyone who says, "I shouldn't eat French fries," or

"I have to get a bite of chocolate" will feel that they have no control over the events. Instead, if you say "I prefer" to leave the food, you will feel more power and less guilt. The term "dieting" should be avoided. Proper nutrition is a permanent lifestyle change. For example, the correct wording is, "I've changed my eating habits" or "I'm eating healthier."

Diets are fattening. Why?

The body needs fat. Our body wants to live, so it stores fat. Removing this amount of fat from the body is not an easy task as the body protects against weight loss. During starvation, our bodies switch to a 'saving flame', burning fewer calories to avoid starving. Those who are starting to lose weight are usually optimistic, as, during the first week, they may experience 1-3 kg (2-7 lbs.) Of weight loss, which validates their efforts and suffering. Their body, however, has deceived them very well because it actually does not want to break down fat. Instead, it begins to break down muscle tissue. At the beginning of dieting, our bodies burn sugar and protein, not fat. Burned sugar removes a lot of water out of the body; that's why we experience amazing results on the scale. It should take about seven days for our body to switch to fat burning. Then our body's alarm bell rings. Most diets have a sad end: reducing your metabolic rate to a lower level—meaning, that if you only eat a little more afterwards, you regain all the weight you have lost previously. After dieting, the body will make special efforts to store fat for the next impending famine. What to do to prevent such a situation?

We must understand what our soul needs. Those who really desire to have success must first and foremost change their spiritual foundation. It is important to pamper our souls during a period of weight loss. All overweight people tend to rag on themselves for eating forbidden food, "I overate again. My willpower is so weak!" If you have ever tried to lose weight, you know these thoughts very well.

Imagine a person very close to you who has gone through a difficult time while making mistakes from time to time. Are we going to scold or try to help and motivate them? If we really love them, we will instead comfort them and try to convince them to continue. No one tells their best friend that they are weak, ugly, or bad, just because they are struggling with their weight. If you wouldn't say it to your friend, don't do so to yourself either! Let us be aware of this: during weight loss, our soul needs peace and support. Realistic thinking is more useful than disaster theory. If you are generally a healthy consumer, eat some goodies sometimes because of its delicious taste and to pamper your soul.

I'll give you a list of a hundred positive affirmations you can use to reinforce your weight loss. I'll divide them into main categories based on the most typical situations for which you would need confirmation. You can repeat all of them whenever you need to, but you can also choose the ones that are more suitable for your circumstances. If you prefer to listen to them during meditation, you can record them with a piece of sweet relaxing music in the background.

General affirmations to reinforce your wellbeing:

1. I'm grateful that I woke up today. Thank you for making me happy today.
2. Today is a perfect day. I meet nice and helpful people, whom I treat kindly.
3. Every new day is for me. I live to make myself feel good. Today I just pick good thoughts for myself.
4. Something wonderful is happening to me today.
5. I feel good.
6. I am calm, energetic and cheerful.
7. My organs are healthy.
8. I am satisfied and balanced.
9. I live in peace and understanding with everyone.
10. I listen to others with patience.
11. In every situation, I find the good.
12. I accept and respect myself and my fellow human beings.
13. I trust myself; I trust my inner wisdom.

Do you often scold yourself? Then repeat the following affirmations frequently:

1. I forgive myself.
2. I'm good to myself.
3. I motivate myself over and over again.
4. I'm doing my job well.
5. I care about myself.
6. I am doing my best.
7. I am proud of myself for my achievements.
8. I am aware that sometimes I have to pamper my soul.
9. I remember that I did a great job this week.
10. I deserved this small piece of candy.
11. I let go of the feeling of guilt.
12. I release the blame.
13. Everyone is imperfect. I accept that I am too.

If you feel pain when you choose to avoid delicious food, then you need to motivate yourself with affirmations such as:

1. I am motivated and persistent.
2. I control my life and my weight.
3. I'm ready to change my life.
4. Changes make me feel better.
5. I follow my diet with joy and cheerfulness.
6. I am aware of my amazing capacities.
7. I am grateful for my opportunities.

8. Today I'm excited to start a new diet.

9. I always keep in mind my goals.

10. I imagine myself slim and beautiful.

11. Today I am happy to have the opportunity to do what I have long been postponing.

12. I possess the energy and will to go through my diet.

13. I prefer to lose weight instead of wasting time on momentary pleasures.

Here you can find affirmations that help you to change harmful convictions and blockages:

1. I see my progress every day.

2. I listen to my body's messages.

3. I'm taking care of my health.

4. I eat healthy food.

5. I love who I am.

6. I love how life supports me.

7. A good parking space, coffee, conversation. It's all for me today.

8. It feels good to be awake because I can live in peace, health, love.

9. I'm grateful that I woke up. I take a deep breath of peace and tranquility.

10. I love my body. I love being served by me.

11. I eat by tasting every flavor of the food.

12. I am aware of the benefits of healthy food.

13. I enjoy eating healthy food and being fitter every day.

14. I feel energetic because I eat well.

Many people are struggling with being overweight because they don't move enough. The very root of this issue can be a refusal to do exercises due to negative biases in our minds.

We can overcome these beliefs by repeating the following affirmations:

1. I like moving because it helps my body burn fat.

2. Each time I exercise, I am getting closer to having a beautiful, tight shapely body.

3. It's a very uplifting feeling of being able to climb up to 100 steps without stopping.

4. It's easier to have an excellent quality of life if I move.

5. I like the feeling of returning to my home tired but happy after a long winter walk.

6. Physical exercises help me have a longer life.

7. I am proud to have better fitness and agility.

8. I feel happier thanks to the happiness hormone produced by exercise.

9. I feel full thanks to the enzymes that produce a sense of fullness during physical exercises.

10. I am aware even after exercise, my muscles continue to burn fat, and so I lose weight while resting.

11. I feel more energetic after exercises.

12. My goal is to lose weight; therefore, I exercise.

13. I am motivated to exercise every day.

14. I lose weight while I exercise.

Now, I am going to give you a list of generic affirmations that you can build in your program:

1. I'm glad I'm who I am.
2. Today, I read articles and watch movies that make me feel positive about my diet progress.
3. I love it when I'm happy.
4. I take a deep breath and exhale my fears.
5. Today I do not want to prove my truth, but I want to be happy.
6. I am strong and healthy. I'm fine, and I'm getting better.
7. I am happy today because whatever I do, I find joy in it.
8. I pay attention to what I can become.
9. I love myself and am helpful to others.
10. I accept what I cannot change.
11. I am happy that I can eat healthy food.
12. I am happy that I have been changing my life with my new healthy lifestyle.
13. Today I do not compare myself to others.
14. I accept and support who I am and turn to myself with love.
15. Today I can do anything for my improvement.
16. I'm fine. I'm happy for life. I love who I am. I'm strong and confident.

17. I am calm and satisfied.

18. Today is perfect for me to exercise and to be healthy.

19. I have decided to lose weight, and I am strong enough to follow my will.

20. I love myself, so I want to lose weight.

21. I am proud of myself because I follow my diet program.

22. I see how much stronger I am.

23. I know that I can do it.

24. It is not my past, but my present that defines me.

25. I am grateful for my life.

26. I am grateful for my body because it collaborates well with me.

27. Eating healthy foods supports me to get the best nutrients I need to be in the best shape.

28. I eat only healthy foods, and I avoid processed foods.

29. I can achieve my weight loss goals.

30. All cells in my body are fit and healthy, and so am I.

31. I enjoy staying healthy and sustaining my ideal weight.

32. I feel that my body is losing weight right now.

33. I care about my body by exercising every day.

Chapter 8: How to Practice Every Day

Exercise Regularly

Exercise is good for human health in many ways, regardless of what you choose to do.

Although the DASH diet focuses on food choices, there is no denying that regular and varied exercise represents an essential component of a healthy lifestyle and one that can confer additional benefits.

With that said, the CDC identifies moderate-intensity aerobic activity that totals 120 to 150 minutes weekly, in combination with two additional weekly days of muscular resistance training, as an ideal combination to confer numerous health benefits to adults. Per the CDC, these benefits include the following:

Better weight management: When combined with dietary modification, regular physical activity plays a role in supporting or enhancing weight-management efforts. Regular exercise is a great way to expend calories on top of any dietary changes you will be making on this program.

Reduced risk for cardiovascular disease: A reduction in blood pressure is a well-recognized benefit of regular physical activity, which ultimately contributes to a reduced risk of cardiovascular disease.

Reduced risk of type 2 diabetes: Regular physical activity is known to improve blood glucose control and insulin sensitivity.

Improved mood: Regular physical activity is associated with improvements in mood and reductions in anxiety owing to how exercise positively influences the biochemistry of the human brain by releasing hormones and affecting neurotransmitters.

Better sleep: Those who exercise more regularly tend to sleep better than those who don't, which may be partly owing to the reductions in stress and anxiety that often occur in those who exercise regularly.

Stronger bones and muscles: Combining cardiovascular and resistance training confers severe benefits to both your bones and your muscles, which keep your body functioning at a high level as you age.

A longer life span: Those who exercise regularly tend to enjoy a lower risk of chronic disease and a longer life span.

As you will see in the 28-day plan, your recommended

exercise totals will meet by exercising four out of the seven days a week. The exercise days will break up as follows: All four of the active days will include aerobic exercise for 30 minutes. As a beginner, I encourage you to start slowly and build up to four days. Two of the four active days will also include strength training. The bottom line is that you don't have to exercise for hours each day to enjoy the health benefits of physical activity. Our goal with this plan is to make the health benefits of exercise as accessible and attainable as possible for those who are ready and willing to give it a try.

Getting the Most Out of Your Workouts

Just as with healthy eating strategies, there are certain essential things to keep in mind about physical activity that will help support your long-term success. Let's take a look at a few crucial considerations that will help you get the most out of your workouts:

Rest days: Even though we haven't even started, I'm going to preach the importance of proper rest. Don't forget that you are taking part in this journey to improve your health for the long term, not to burn yourself out in 28 days. Although some of you with more experience with exercise may feel confident going above and beyond, my best advice for the majority of those reading is to listen to your body and take days off to minimize the risk of injury and burnout.

Stretching life: Stretching is a great way to prevent injury and keep your pain-free both during workouts and daily. Whether it's a planned activity after an exercise or through additional means such as yoga, stretching is beneficial in many ways.

Enjoyment: There is no right or wrong style of exercise. You are being provided with a different plan that emphasizes a variety of different cardiovascular and resistance training exercises. If there are certain activities within these groups that you don't enjoy, it's okay not to do them. Your ability to stick with regular physical activity in the long term will depend on finding a style of exercise that you enjoy.

Your limits: Physical activity is right for you, and it should be fun, too. It's up to you to keep it that way. While it is essential to challenge yourself, don't risk injury by taking things too far too fast.

Your progress: Although this is not an absolute requirement, some of you reading may find joy and fulfilment through tracking your exercise progress and striving toward a longer duration, more repetitions, and so on. If you are the type who enjoys a competitive edge, it may be fun to find a buddy to exercise and progress with.

Warm-ups: Last but certainly not least, your exercise routine will benefit significantly from a proper warm-up routine, which includes starting slowly or doing exercises similar to the ones included in your workout, but at a lower intensity.

Set a Routine

The exercise part of the DASH plan was developed with CDC exercise recommendations in mind to support your best health. For some, the 28-day policy may seem like a lot; for others, it may not seem like that much. If we look at any exercise routine from a very general perspective, there are at least three broad categories to be aware of.

Strength training: This involves utilizing your muscles against some form of counterweight, which may be your own body or dumbbells. These types of activities alter your resting metabolic rate by supporting the development of muscle while also strengthening your bones.

Aerobic exercise: Also known as a cardiovascular activity, these are the quintessential exercises such as jogging or running that involve getting your body moving and getting your heart rate up.

Mobility, flexibility, and balance: Stretching after workouts or even devoting your exercise time on one day a week to stretching or yoga is a great way to maintain mobility and prevent injury in the long term.

This routine recommends involving a combination of both cardiovascular and resistance training.

You will be provided with a wide array of options to choose from to accommodate a diverse exercise routine.

My best recommendation is to settle on the types of exercises that offer a balance between enjoyment and challenge. Remember that the benefits of physical activity are to be enjoyed well beyond just your 28-day plan, and the best way to ensure that is the case is selecting movements you genuinely enjoy.

Cardio and Body Weight Exercises

Running: The quintessential and perhaps most well-recognized cardiovascular exercise.

Jumping jacks: Although 30 minutes straight of jumping jacks may be impractical, they are an excellent complement to the other activities on this list.

Dancing: Those who have a background in dancing may enjoy using it to their advantage, but anyone can put on their favorite songs and dance like there's nobody watching.

Jump rope: Own a jump rope? Why not use it as part of your cardiovascular workout? It is a fun way to get your cardio in.

Other options (equipment permitting): Activities like rowing, swimming and water aerobics, biking, and using elliptical and stair climbing machines can be great ways to exercise.

With the guidelines, your goal will be to work up to a total of 30 minutes of cardiovascular activity per workout session. You may use a combination of the exercises listed. I suggest that beginners should start with brisk walking or jogging— whatever activity you are most comfortable with.

Core

Plank: The plank is a classic core exercise that focuses on the stability and strength of the muscles in the abdominal and surrounding areas. Engage your buttocks, press your forearms into the ground, and hold for 60 seconds. Beginners may start with a 15- to 30-second hold and work their way up.

Side plank: Another core classic and a plank variation that focuses more on the oblique muscles on either side of your central abdominals. Keep the buttocks tight and prevent your torso from sagging to get the most out of this exercise.

Woodchopper: A slightly more dynamic movement that works the rotational functionality of your core and mimics chopping a log of wood. You can start with little to no weight until you feel comfortable and progress from there. Start the move with feet shoulder-width apart, back straight, and slightly crouched. If you are using weight, hold it with both hands next to the outside of either thigh, twist to the side, and lift the weight across and upward, keeping your arms straight and turning your torso such that you end up with the weight above your opposite shoulder.

Lower Body

Goblet squat: Start your stance with feet slightly wider than shoulder-width and a dumbbell held tightly with both hands in front of your chest. Sit back into a squat, hinging at both the knee and the hip joint, and lower your legs until they are parallel to the ground. Push up through your heels to the starting position and repeat. Use a chair to squat onto if you don't feel comfortable.

Dumbbell walking lunge: Start upright with a dumbbell in each hand and feet in your usual standing position. Step forward with one leg and sink until your back knee is just above the ground. Remain upright and ensure the front knee does not bend over the toes. Push through the heel of the front foot and step forward and through with your rear foot.

Start with no weights and add weight as you feel comfortable.

Upper Body

Push-ups: These are the ultimate body-weight exercise and can be done just about anywhere. You will want to set up with your hands just beyond shoulder width, keeping your body in a straight line and always engaging your core as you ascend and descend, without letting your elbows flare out. Those who struggle to perform push-ups consecutively can start by performing them on their knees or even against a wall if regular push-ups sound like too much.

Dumbbell shoulder press: An excellent exercise for upper-body and shoulder strength. Bring a pair of dumbbells to ear level, palms forward, and straighten your arms overhead.

Full Body

Mountain climbers: On your hands and feet, keep your body in a straight line, with your abdominal and buttocks muscles engaged, similar to the top position of a push-up. Rapidly alternate pulling your knees into your chest while keeping your core tight. Continue in this left, right, left, right rhythm as if you are replicating a running motion. Always try to keep your spine in a straight line.

Push press: This is essentially a combination move incorporating a partial squat and a dumbbell shoulder press. Using a weight that you are comfortable with, stand feet slightly beyond shoulder width, with light dumbbells held in a pressing position. Descend for a squat to a depth you feel comfortable with, and on the ascent simultaneously push the dumbbells overhead.

Chapter 9: Additional Tips for Weight Loss

Understanding Habit

If you try to make a difference in your life, you're working to alter old habits and to create new ones. Sitting down and thinking about the improvements you want in your life is easy, but they are hard to execute and keep going. It's because you've produced patterns that need to be changed to be successful.

I have taught a lot of customers in my career, and almost every customer I teach knows what they have to do to achieve their target, but they can't. How do you do that?

Since they don't choose to take the necessary action periodically to develop habits that will produce long-term results.

Our customs control our actions. Understanding habits and their role in your life is essential, as they are responsible for your daytime choices. An individual does not lose weight because he or she is not aware that during commercial breaks, he or she is used to going to the kitchen to eat. For some instances, habit is something we don't know about. We do so consciously. Being mindful of your habits gives you the strength to make your life-changing decision. It's hard to make a decision when you know what your options are.

It's essential to be mindful of your old habits and the new ones you need to create while you are making changes in your life. Just think about the change you'd like to make. (Lose weight, get in shape, and get more energy) Now think about where you are right now, and what shift you want to make. (Lose 30 lbs., have more stamina, build strength, have more energy) Now think about the past and the acts you've taken, which are responsible for where you're at. (Eat fast food, watch TV, and drink too much every night).

Now ask yourself what actions do I need to take to bring about the change that I want to see in my life? The solutions you'll come up with are the acts you need to turn into behaviors. A habit is something you do, and you do not worry about it. You need to do the behavior regularly to build this habit before you have to think about it.

Habits aren't instantly created. It's something you have to do, consistently, for an extended period. How long does it take to do this? When you do it, and you do not have to worry about it. I read a lot of different stuff about how long it takes to build a habit ... Thirty days, sixty, ninety days ... I think these are fantastic goals, but I know it may take you a little longer. If this is a move that you want to make, you're going to do the research and work hard to make it happen.

Habits can be divided into two categories: motor and (actually) mental habits.

We reflect daily ways of acting or thinking we know without grappling with our will or even voluntary strength. Habits are acquired by learning, and then particularly by repetition.

It is, therefore, essential that the components (acts or thoughts) be replicated regularly and several times until a new habit is created.

Running, walking, walking, driving and so on are things that we had to know.

When we understand habits, we usually think of the behavior we replicate, and the habit of science will tell us why we replicate our patterns and develop habits as we grow up.

Habits are also repeated patterns of actions and behaviors that we are conditioned to perform, and that can evolve over many years, and habits that have evolved over many years are more likely to be stronger than those that have been developed recently or in a few years.

And habits that we learn as children remain with us all our lives are more likely than habits that we learn as adults. And the frequency or success of those habits would be directly linked to how long we have had those patterns of behavior.

And this is the routine that we all formed as children waking up in the morning and brushing our teeth. Now we have to wonder what if we're trying to stop the habits? What if we wake up and have not brushed our teeth? Besides the fact that we can end up with bad breath when we don't obey one of our everyday routines, there are real psychological effects of physical and emotional or social distress!

Brushing your teeth is a case in point. Another could be when you enter your apartment and turn on the TV or computer shortly after you return home. In your immediate area, you immediately feel uncomfortable if you stop doing so, even if it's your own home, as though something is missing from your life.

Suppose your TV or laptop is broken down, you can't exercise the habit, and you feel depressed. We, humans, are slaves to these patterns of behavior, and thus habits are an important part of our lives. This discomfort we feel can be seen as the product of 'habit obstruction' when we are unable to exercise our habits. Thus, the effects of disruption of habit may have a significant effect on our emotional, social and personal lives.

If habit obstruction effect is long-term, that is when your

laptop is broken for weeks or months. You can't turn it on when you enter your house or apartment, and the habit obstruction effect will spread to habit hunger. After a few weeks of habit obstruction, you may even start losing your habit subconsciously when you get into the habit hunger effect.

So, habit hunger can cause some form of amnesia from your usual behavior, and you forget about that habit. It's all very good, but then not so simple, because you might have some form of habit displacement in this case and develop some other habit.

The Importance of Habits

Behind every habit, there is a real need that you need to satisfy. Be it any kind of habit, good or bad. Like for example:

· Who smokes to relieve stress?

· Who drinks to relax?

· Whoever exercises for pleasure?

All of these activities, whether harmful or not, contain a yearning for fulfilment for those who practice. This is what makes a habit so challenging to change.

So much so that when trying to change a habit, you will

experience great difficulty in the first few weeks.

Because, when you stop doing something that was already customary, your body will begin to crave that sensation caused by that old custom that you left behind.

Tips to improve your habits

Life is full of habits, good and bad, it is just as easy to have positive habits as negative, but transforming them implies an effort and a lot of willpower, a change of beliefs and appreciation.

The answer is in you, can you change your habits?

·   Know the habits you would like to adopt. Start by making a detailed list of the habits you would like to change or improve.

·   Analyze the attitudes that general conflicts. If you have not been able to identify all the bad habits or do not think you do not have them, ask yourself what kind of behaviors generate conflicts in your daily life and with the people around you, an example would be if you arrive at your appointments late and this causes discomfort in other people if you have no energy because you do not eat healthily or if you are a little overweight and you dislike it.

·   Become aware of the importance of changing bad habits.

It is important to raise awareness subtly to the people closest to you about the importance of improving their habits. If they do it simultaneously, it will be easier to adopt them. For example, if someone in your family buys junk food and you are looking for a healthy diet, it is vital to encourage them not to do so that everyone improves their habits and their diet, especially if this person is overweight.

· Build an action plan. Once you have identified the habits you would like to adopt, you need to make an action plan to carry it out. The first step is to become aware of the habit you want to change and continuously monitor your actions and thinking patterns to identify why you react that way. The next thing will be to repeat the new habit every day for at least 30 days, and it is the minimum time in which a habit is adopted. For example, if you want to start exercising, do it at least four days a week for two months. In this way, your body and mind will adapt to the new activities you do.

· Be honest with yourself. Finally, you must be objective and recognize if you have continued repeating the new habits, analyze if you already feel that they are part of your daily life. If not, it is important to examine the causes that prevented you from achieving it.

Habits are nothing more than the daily repetition of an attitude and discipline. The best day to start changing your habits is today. If you stop to think about all the time it takes to change a habit, and you probably won't, the important thing is to be determined and start today.

How to Improve Your Eating Habits for Weight Loss

The barriers people have reached for themselves seem to have no end in sight. Hunger, fruit diets and uncooked foods are among the drastic alternatives to the long old weight-loss problem. I had attempted to try these for myself, and none of them succeeded until I closed the diet and only changed my weight loss eating habits.

The diets are similar to weight loss band-aids. In a short-term illness, they are a fast solution and do not change behavior, metabolism or produce a true bang on body fat. Dictary rigidity does not increase the element of success; in reality, it decreases it. It is much easier to make gradual changes that are not upsetting or penalizing but launch the body on the road to equilibrium and its normal set point to some extent. Stable changes in eating habits are certainly an excellent option for losing weight.

Rather than eliminating calories by the end of the day or for a big meal, five or six small food portions are much healthier for the body. This sounds contradictory but real. The body burns calories in everyday exercise. This requires food calories to feed and digest. Reports show that up to 10% of calories are used to process the food.

Therefore, 50 calories are needed for food processing for a 500-calorie serving. It's been shown that eating less often helps in weight gain over the long term. To strengthen your weight-loss eating habits, you will regularly consume yet healthy foods. A psychosomatic eating benefit is feeling good. The feeling you're not hollow is beneficial in continuing the weight loss cycle.

Booming weight loss isn't a major science, nor does it entail difficulty and pain—easy changes like cooking nutritious meals 5-6 times a day. Eating the right part size is critical. Eating the right calories is important, and daily exercise is important. Eat and consume the right form of food are the safest dietary habits for weight loss.

Chapter 10: Love Your Body and Your Soul

Glad individuals acknowledge and love themselves regardless of what their body resembles, irrespective of how they feel. An ideal organization isn't preferred or all the more empowering over a body not considered immaculate by the "powers that be." Your magnificence originates from inside.

Consider somebody you know (or knew) who isn't generally all that appealing; however, who appears to adore herself so much that she feels delightful and acts as needs be. Individuals like that tend to be well known. Curiously, their excellence sparkles so splendidly that they seem, by all accounts, to be alluring to others.

Individuals in the media don't typically seem as though they seem to look in front of an audience or magazines and films. That is the reason the calling of make-up specialists exists. In my mind, what they do is make-up how this individual will appear to the crowd and fans. When photograph distributing is included, nobody is viewed as they look. All pictures get finished up.

At the point when you love yourself, honestly and genuinely

love yourself, regardless of how old you develop to be your sentiments about you won't change. The fascinating piece about adoring yourself is living in a condition of satisfaction. Hardly any individuals get the chance to abide there—the individuals who do remain youthful until the end of time.

Tips to Assist You with Adoring Your Body

1. Take power back to characterize your Beauty

You are not just taking it back for the social/media definitions yet in addition to individuals around you in your life who have offered critical comments about your body. These individuals couldn't see the magnificence of your body since they had retained the standard definitions themselves and were deciding for you and most likely their body against these gauges too. Pause for a minute presently to close your eyes and envision reclaiming the power to characterize the excellence of your body. Take it once again from the social definitions and the media in your mental state, "I won't permit you to characterize what my body ought to resemble any longer." Think back to individuals that had offered negative remarks to you about your body a relative, a sentimental accomplice, or different children when you were close to nothing. State to them in your mind, "I reclaim the power to characterize the magnificence of my body your remarks were bends and false, and I no longer give them any power." Feel how great this feels to free yourself from the entirety of this cynicism.

2. Clear Your Negative Beliefs about Your Body

Due to your introduction to the social molding about the alleged perfect female body you presumably have rehearsed self-judgment of your body for not fitting in with the advanced "perfect." These decisions and negative convictions are again contortions and not founded on the reality of the one of your very kind stunner body. We, as a whole, have groups of various sizes and shapes that are uncommon and genuinely delightful.

Relinquish your unbending convictions about how your body should look and start to perceive how the very things that are diverse about your body are the very things that make you one of a kind and lovely. Record the negative messages that you state to yourself about your body. Envision thinking of them to discharge them from your cognizance. Get them hard and fast, the most negative terrible ones you can consider. Take a gander at these messages, notice how you could never fantasy about directing these sentiments toward any other person in your life. Take a gander at all of these messages and apologize to your body, saying, "I'm sorry to such an extent that I directed these harmful sentiments toward you, I guarantee that I won't direct these sentiments toward you again and I will begin adoring you." Look at these messages again and with an expectation to completely discharge them destroy the piece of paper and discard it. A few people like to fabricate a fire outside and consume the document as a method of releasing this cynicism.

3. Exercise for the Joy of Feeling Your Body Move

At the point when you exercise to take out fat from your body as well as to make up for calories, eaten this can emerge out of a position of fear and have a vitality of attempting to control and battle against your body. Envision practicing for the delight of moving your body and from a goal to be wanting to your body, a craving for it to be sound and have more vitality. The customers I work with around this issue will, in general, have the option to keep up an activity program if they do it from a position of satisfaction and self-love as opposed to control and fear about their weight.

Notice if there are things throughout your life that you don't accomplish for fear of individuals seeing your body, like swimming, moving, or any other movement. Remind yourself that you have the right to do the things you appreciate regardless of your shape. Relinquish what others consider you and remain concentrated on the way that you reserve each option to do the things you understand.

4. Remind Yourself What the Purpose of Having a Body Is

Your body is yours to encounter life; ultimately, to take it in and appreciate it. Your body is a vehicle for you to encounter existence with the entirety of your faculties. Your body permits you: to feel a warm breeze on your skin, feel the cold water in a lake when you swim, see the entirety of the striking shades of nightfall, hear the whole of the excellence of the music, to listen to the hints of fowls and trees moving in the breeze, feel the non-abrasiveness of somebody's hand, feel the delight of moving, taste and appreciate flavorful food, communicate through a grin, tears or giggling. Your body is for you, for nobody else to investigate or pass judgment. You are not here as a presentation for other people; however, as a wholly encapsulated person with more profound, more extravagant characteristics than merely your appearance.

5. at the point when you look in The Mirror-Look at Yourself through Loving Eyes

For some, ladies glancing in the mirror transforms into an activity of self-judgment. They focus on the entirety of their apparent flaws and what they feel is "off-base" with their body or face. Again, the models they are deciding for themselves against is this ridiculous perfect that is advanced in the media. I have numerous customers who, when they previously began working with me, said that they couldn't glance in the mirror since all they saw were these apparent flaws. I recommend that they move this by instead taking a gander at themselves in the mirror through adoring eyes. A model would be if you look in the mirror and see a wrinkle that you would generally judge, see this wrinkle with affection and empathy and even observe the excellence of this wrinkle. Set an away from to see yourself through the perspective of adoration intrude on the self-judgment and move into being exceptionally cherishing with yourself. This will be something that you have to rehearse before it turns into a propensity. Yet, it will be justified even despite the exertion since you will start to feel extremely magnificent about yourself.

6. Have Your Self-Esteem be Internally Referenced

Have your self-regard be founded on your interior characteristics as opposed to your outside appearance. What are the features that make yourself you? Is it your sympathy, your new innovativeness, your insight, your ability to have a ton of fun, your awareness, your perceptiveness, your ability to tune in to individuals, or your caring heart? Think about the individuals that you love in your life. You love them for what their identity is, the one of a kind Spirit that they are, not for what they resemble. That is how they feel about you, they love you for what your identity is and the entirety of the extraordinary characteristics that make up you. Figure out how to esteem yourself for the substance of you, not for the physical structure that you travel around in.

7. Investigate the deeper purpose behind the distraction with your appearance/weight.

Here and there, when somebody is engrossed with their appearance, it might be a shirking system for more profound, increasingly agonizing sentiments. Check-in with yourself and check whether this may be the situation. If in your youth things were excruciating for you and crazy, you may have figured out how to concentrate on your weight as an approach to keep away from the forlornness and defenselessness of what was going on around you. Or then again, perhaps there is a problematic issue in your life today that you don't have the fearlessness to confront like a problematic relationship or absence of direction in your life. A distraction with your appearance occupies you from facing these issues. If so, for you, it is significant for you to get support for yourself to open up to confront these sentiments straightforwardly. You can get this help through facing the challenge to uncover your feelings to a confided in companion or working with an advocate who can assist you with working through these emotions.

8. Take out Comparing Yourself to Others

The vitality of correlation and rivalry is damaging to yourself and the other individual. Doing this is simply one more type of putting yourself and won't help you to feel better; however, it will exacerbate you think even. Pledge to pass on this sort of vitality. Instead, if you see somebody who is appealing as opposed to contrasting yourself with this individual or making a decision about them, the state instead, "She is alluring as am I." Celebrate that other individual and yourself as well. You will discover this feels such a significant amount of superior to contrasting yourself with them or being basic.

9. Take One of the Areas of Your Body You Typically Judge and Take a Week to Fully Love This Part of You

Go through 15 minutes daily taking a gander at this piece of your body, and discover things to adore about it, even better, do it for the day. The additionally testing it is to do this, the more you have to do it! I read in a book about a lady who did this activity, and following seven days of doing it, an outsider came up to her and revealed to her how delightful this piece of her body was! At the point when we change our particular manner of seeing ourselves, it changes the style in which others see us as well. You need your first expectation of doing this activity to be simply the move in your affection, not to have an impact on how others see you. How you see you are continually going to be what is generally significant.

Conclusion

Let's look back at our progress and then paying it forward to others. Continue eating better all day. You'll feel better, look better, achieve your goals, and have a better quality of life. Assuming you've read and understood all the content here, chances are that you've realized your habits and applying core solutions to overcoming obstacles while holding yourself accountable, you have Paid attention to yourself, your purpose, unique talents, and dreams. By automating your food and water, cutting out unhealthy sugar, alcohol and white carbs, adding protein, Greek yogurt or other probiotics, produce and healthy fats.

Choose to continue with the same eating habit all your life. Focus on a healthy weight; stay with silence. Visualize your step and take steps that are going to get you to where you want to be. If you destabilize procrastination, stress and comfort zone, you will go farther at a fast pace. Organize your kitchen and automate your food. Be a reader; Read positive affirmations aloud every day. Pursue your goals, including your fitness and health goals that will utilize your talents and passions and keep you on the healthy-fit journey. Rest on weekends and follow the process again.

Focus on your activities, journalize your progress, thoughts, and move on. Record your success, nature; they will guide you in thinking and solving stress, among other problems. You will make not only an impact on yourself but also the people around you. Make use of productivity apps on the internet to guide you through.

While writing your journal, consider how you've grown physically, mentally, spiritually, and emotionally or socially. Think about how one area has positively affected other areas. If some things haven't worked out for you, spend some time forgiving other people, forgiving yourself so you can move on. Giving makes living worthwhile.

Albert Einstein believed that a life shared with others is worthy. We have people out there who need you, remember not to hoard your successes. Share your success. Share your new-found recipes, your attitude, and your habits. Share what you have learned with others. In all your undertakings, know that you can't change other people but yourself, therefore, be mindful. Reflect on your changes and put yourself on the back today and every day. Be grateful and live your life as a champion.

Make it a reality on your mind, the fact that the journey to a healthy life and weight loss is long and has many challenges. Pieces of Stuff we consider more important in life require our full cooperation towards them. Just because you are facing problems in your Wight loss journey, it does not mean that you should stop, instead show and prove the whole world how good your ability to handle constant challenges is—training your brain to know that eating healthy food together with functional exercises can work miracles. Make it your choice and not something you are forced to do by a third party. Always tell yourself that weight loss is a long process and not an event. Take every day of your days to celebrate your achievements because these achievements are what piles up to a massive victory. Make a list of stuff you would like to change when you get healthy they may be Small size-clothes, being able to accumulate enough energy, participating in your most loved sports you have been admiring for a more extended period, feeling self-assured. Make these tips your number one source of empowerment; you will end up completing your 30 days even without noticing.

You have made it, or you are about to make it. The journey has been unbelievable. And by now, you must be having a story to tell. Concentrate on finishing strongly. Keep up the excellent eating design you have adopted. Remember, you are not working on temporary changes but long-term goals. Therefore, lifestyle changes should not be stopped when the weight is lost. Remind yourself always of essential habits that are easier to follow daily. They include trusting yourself and the process by acknowledging that the real change lies in your hands. Stop complacency, arise, and walk around for at least thirty minutes away. Your breakfast is the most important meal you deserve. Eat your breakfast like a queen. For each diet, you take, add a few proteins and natural fats. Let hunger not kill you, eat more, but just what is recommended, bring snacks and other meals 3 or 5 times a day. Have more veggies and fruits like 5-6 rounds in 24 hours. Almost 90% of Americans do not receive enough vegetables and fruits to their satisfaction. Remember, Apple will not make you grow fat. Substitute salt. You will be shocked by the sweet taste of food once you stop consuming salt. Regain your original feeling, you will differentiate natural flavorings from artificial flavors. Just brainstorm how those older adults managed to eat their food without salt or modern-day characters. Characters are not suitable for your health. Drink a lot of water in a day. Let water be your number one drink. Avoid soft drinks and other energy drinks, and they are slowly killing you. Drink a lot of water in the morning after getting out of your bed. Your body will be fresh from morning to evening. Have a journal and be realistic with it. Take charge of what you write and be responsible.

CPSIA information can be obtained
at www.ICGtesting.com
Printed in the USA
BVHW040806070321
601819BV00021B/227

9 781801 779852